Weight Loss

20+ Healthy Snacks To Lose Weight Fast

Table of content

Introduction

Losing weight is no easy task. There are so many things that must be considered, that it can be overwhelming. You need to pick a diet, find an exercise plan, and actually go through with it. Nobody can do that all by themselves, and there are a plethora of resources on the Internet, in person, and more for you to utilize. But one of the most trusted name in weight loss is Weight Watchers. They have helped generations of men and women take control of their problems with food, weight loss, and exercise plans. Celebrities have endorsed their program, and shared their success stories with the world. By following a weight watchers diet plan, you give yourself a much better chance of being successful in reaching your weight loss goals.

However, even in picking and sticking with a diet, it can be difficult. Diet plans will give you general guidelines with what foods to pick and oftentimes leave the foods you should be eating for snacks vague. Finding exact meals and recipes to eat for meals and snacks alike can be difficult after a time, as the recipes that you know are healthy begin to become boring, and you want a change.

With snacks, this desire for something new and better does not change. We enjoy our favorites, and we fall back on these, but sometimes we need a change. In order to even find our favorite snacks and foods, we need to explore. Through this book, hopefully you will find your new favorites, and add to the snacks that you add to your regular routine.

Through this book, we hope to show you the different ways that you can spice up your nutritional playbook. It is separated into four different chapters, each with a general theme and distinguishing ingredient. The chapters are based off of snacks that highlight vegetables and fruit. It is always important to get at least seven serving of fruit and vegetables in your diet. Vegetables are much harder to fit into diets, because many people do not like the taste. But the snacks in this book will take the healthy nature of vegetables, and make them delicious, without making them unhealthy by breading them and frying them. Vegetables do not have the be the hardest part of your diet any longer.

Fruits are much easier to incorporate into your diet, because they are sweeter, and it is easier to find a taste and flavor that suits anyone's flavor palate. However, fruits have natural sugars, and need to be made in the right quantities, and paired with the right foods in order to remain healthy.

The next two chapters will be based on more substantial meal ideas. The chapter on desserts will take the best and most decadent desserts that one could possibly think of, but find ways to make them healthier, and in a smaller portion that can be more easily added into your daily caloric intake. This is where we will show you how to take things like strawberry cheesecake, and make them healthy, and smaller portioned.

The final chapter will be based on decadent and unhealthy foods that we have revamped for the best overall taste, while remaining healthy. It is in this chapter that you can find foods such as onion rings, and meatballs. Just because it is healthy, does not mean that it has to be disgusting.

Chapter 1 – Vegetable Snacks

Southwestern Kale Chips

One of the best ways to add more vegetables into your life and find a replacement for potato chips is to try kale chips. I know, it sounds gross, but before you completely disregard it, read the recipe and see for yourself how easily kale can be transformed into an intimidating vegetable, into a delectable and addicting snack.

You will need to tear one bunch of kale into pieces that are around the same size as a potato chip, put them on the side. In a bowl, you will need to add olive oil, apple cider vinegar, salt, garlic powder, ground cumin, chili powder, cayenne pepper, and black pepper together, combining them together before adding the kale into the mix, coating each piece in the mixture. Replace the kale on the cookie sheet, and cook the kale at 275 degrees for about 20 minutes, making sure to slip the leaves after 10 minutes.

Once the timer is complete, allow the kale chips to rest on a paper towel to cool down, and enjoy! They can be easily stored in a Ziploc bag to store them for later.

Avocado Dip

Guacamole is one of the most popular dips, for good reason. It is versatile, full of flavor, and packed with nutrients. However, in order to maximize flavor while retaining nutrition, you need to right recipe. Following these instructions will give you the best game day snack, or mid-day munchies satisfaction. Avocados are considered healthy fats, and can help you build up the good cholesterol in your body that is necessary for your body to function properly, and is the highlight of this meal.

The first step is to peel and seed two avocados, and mash them in a bowl. Adding lime juice, tomato, jalapeno, garlic, cilantro, plain fat free Greek yogurt, cumin, black pepper and salt, combine together until the mixture has a smooth and uniform consistency.

From here, you can serve it fresh and ready to go, or it can be easily refrigerated and stored when ready to go. It can be paired with anything, from carrots and bell peppers, to pita chips to even the kale chips that we just made in the previous recipe.

Spinach Artichoke Dip

Dips are the easiest ways to snack, because they can be paired with a variety of dipping materials, and is easily stored and transported to work, school, or anywhere else your busy life takes you. You can make this spinach artichoke dip on the weekend, and use it throughout your week as a quick fix snack that will satisfy your hunger and your taste buds at the same time.

In order to achieve maximum flavor, wrap onion and garlic in aluminum foil and bake for 20 to 30 minutes until soft in 350 degree oven. While that is cooking, wash and dry spinach, and place in a food processor or blender and pulse it to chop it. Then, combine the cooked garlic and onion, artichoke hearts, tofu, lemon juice, kosher salt, black pepper, and cayenne pepper together, and blend together until it reaches the consistency that you are satisfied with. Making your own healthy spinach artichoke dip is quick and easy! You can then pair this with freshly made kale chips, vegetables, and homemade tortilla chips.

Stuffed Mushrooms

When you think healthy food, how often do mushrooms come to mind? Probably not very often, as they are often eclipsed by foods like kale and spinach and pomegranates, which are much more fad. Mushrooms can be strong sources of B12, and have been shown to help protect your immune system, as well as defend your cardiovascular health and fight cancer. They are a wonderful ingredient to add into any dish, but can be spectacular when served on their own. Stuffed mushrooms is an easy snack that can be enjoyed by all.

First you must clean your cremini mushrooms with a damp paper towel and remove the stems, but save the stems. You should mince the stems, and put them to the side. Sauté garlic in a pan with extra virgin olive oil, and add the stems of the mushrooms, and shallots, and let them cook. Add the parsley, and turn off the heat. In another pan, make a rue with olive oil and flour, whisking the entire time. Add milk slowly, stirring constantly once again. Now, add the nutmeg, salt, and Parmesan cheese to the mixture, and allow it to cool. At this point you can add the egg yolk and the stem mixture, and combined. Fill your mushrooms, and add a sprinkle of breadcrumbs to top before baking in an oven for 20 minutes at 400 degrees.

Cucumber and Tomato Salad

During the warm summer months, who doesn't want a nice cool, refreshing snack? But many of the snacks we turn too are bad and unhealthy for us, and definitely do not follow our diets. What can we do instead? One of the easiest ways to add a refreshing snack, is the cucumber and tomato salad. It is a light snack that will not weigh heavily in your body, but is still delicious and satisfying to enjoy. And the best part about it, it that it is beyond easy to quickly make this meal with few ingredients.

The salad is exceptionally easy to make, all it takes is a quick cutting and combination of cucumbers, tomatoes, and onions, through into a bowl. But what is a salad without a dressing? This dressing is made with Dijon mustard, extra virgin olive oil, balsamic vinegar, fresh dill, salt and black pepper. Combine all of these ingredients, and pour over your salad. For those who find this dressing to tart, you can add a splash of either honey or pure maple syrup, as suits your taste.

Sweet Potato Fries

You will be hard pressed to find someone who says that they do not like French fries. It almost seems like a universal truth, that French fries are a must have with hamburgers, summer nights, and all around tasty goodness. But unfortunately for us, French fries are loaded with bad fats and sodium that our bodies should not be consuming. However, you can swap out your beloved French fries for these delicious and satisfying oven baked sweet potato fries. They turn out just as crispy as addicting as normal French fries, without all of the junk that ends up clogging your heart and weighing your health down overall.

In order to make these, slice your sweet potatoes into the proper size of fry, peeling the skin as you prefer. In a Ziploc bag, combine the potatoes with chili powder, cumin, black pepper, salt, cayenne pepper and olive oil, and combine. You want each of the fries to be coated in the space and olive oil mixture. Line your fries up on a cookie sheet, and back for half an hour at 425 degrees, flipping the fries over after 15 minutes. The spices on these fries can be altered as necessary for different tastes.

Chapter 2 – Snacks with Fruits

Baked Apple Chips

When you get tired of eating vegetables, or if you want a sweater tasting snack to replace your potato chip addiction, baked apple chips can be the best option. They are easy to make, and are only 32 calories in total. It is a simple two-ingredient recipe, which almost everyone has in their homes already.

All that is needed to make these apple chips are apples and cinnamon. It's that simple! First core the apple, and thinly slice the apple. The thinner the slice, the more even the apples will bake. Spread the apples on a cookie sheet that has a layer of parchment paper, and sprinkle cinnamon on top of the apples. Bake in the oven for 275 degrees for two hours, flipping them over after one hour. After you flip the apple slices, it is advised to check on the apples every half an hour so that they do not burn. Once you take them out of the oven, allow them to cool, and then enjoy!

Berry and Quinoa Crisp Parfait

For a refreshing and filling snack, the berry and quinoa crisp parfait is perfect. It combines yogurt, fresh berries, and a crisp quinoa crisp to keep you full and satisfied. For hot days where all you want is something refreshing, but full of the flavors of summer, this snack exceeds expectations. Berries will give you the taste of summer, but quinoa will add a new texture to the snack. You can easily eat this snack during any part of the day, between breakfast and lunch, or even as a dessert snack.

In one bowl, you will need to combine yogurt, honey, and lemon juice. In another pot, add quinoa and water, boiling and then seducing to a simmer, cooking the quinoa for 15 minutes. At this point you can add the honey mixture to the quinoa. Spread the quinoa on a cookie sheet with parchment paper, ensuring that it is spread evenly. Bake for 15 minutes at 325 degrees, and then stir the quinoa. Add an additional 10 minutes of cooking time before layering with yogurt and berries in a bowl.

Chocolate Covered Strawberries

Most people can agree that one of the most decadent foods that they can think of are chocolate covered strawberries. They ooze luxury and are sinfully delicious. But they are often loaded with sugars and calories that can wreck your diet. However, with this recipe, you will maximize the vitamins C and E in strawberries, and the antioxidant powers of chocolate without overloading the snack with calories.

It only takes strawberries, dark chocolate chips, and coconut oil to make. You will need to add a half of a cup to the bottom double boiler, and bring to a simmer. Add the dark chocolate chips as well as the coconut oil to the top boiler, and stir until the chocolate is melted. Remove the chocolate from the heat. Line a cookie sheet with parchment paper and then dip the strawberries into the chocolate, holding onto the leaf, and set on the cookie sheet. You can also add either almond pieces or dried coconut shreds onto the chocolate strawberries immediately after dipping. Allow the strawberries at least 30 minutes to set, and then you can enjoy!

Raspberry Oat Bars

When you go into the store, there are dozens of different kinds of fruit bars, all of which are marketed to be healthy and better for you. They can be eaten as a snack, or as a dessert. But when you begin to look at the nutrition values, and the ingredients list, you find that they are not as healthy as they portray. However, that does not mean that you have to cut fruit bars out of your life. These raspberry oat bars are satisfying, while remaining healthy and low calorie.

You will need to mix white whole wheat flour, rolled oats, coconut palm sugar, baking powder and sea salt, thoroughly mixing them together. Then, add the coconut oil and combine. Spread half of this mixture onto the bottom of a square baking dish, and spreading a fruit sweetened raspberry jam over the mixture. Cover the jam with the other half of the dough, and bake for 25-30 minutes at 350 degrees. Let cool, and then cut into squares before eating.

Dried Fruit

One of the best fruit based snacks that can be easily added into your dietary routine, and is very easy to make, is dried fruit. You can buy dried fruit from stores, but you do not know what else has been done to the fruit to preserve them, whereas with homemade dried fruit, you know exactly how it is made. You can add dried fruit to any meal or snack, or enjoy it on its own. You can use any fruit that you enjoy, with these simple steps.

Whichever fruit you pick must be ripe, but not too ripe. You must wash and peel the fruit, removing any pits and cores, before cutting them into the thickness that you desire. When cutting, make sure to keep the thickness uniform all around to ensure even cooking. Place the fruit slices on a baking sheet, with no pieces touching each other. Cook until the fruit appears dry at 170 degrees, leaving the oven door slightly open, and stirring the fruit every half an hour. Allow the fruit to stand overnight, and then store and enjoy at your leisure.

Peanut Butter Honey Dip with Apple Slices

Dips are clearly one of the best foods to have as a snack. It can be made in large batches and used for several days, saving you time on prep time for all of your meals, and allowing easy access to healthy snacks when you find yourself hungry. This peanut better honey dip with apple slices is one of the best ways that you can add a sweet touch to your snacks, while getting vital nutrients and vitamins into your diet.

You can partner the dip with any fruit that you like, but apples tend to work the best. This dip can also be applied on toast, and added to other meals and ingredients to step up any snack. You need to combine only vanilla Greek yogurt, peanut butter and honey. That is it! Add these ingredients, mixing them together, and refrigerate until it is cool. You can add in cinnamon for additional taste, and chia seeds for additional protein. Dip in apples and any other fruit into the dip and enjoy.

Chapter 3 – Dessert Snacks

Strawberry Cheesecakes

One of the most popular desserts is the cheesecake. It comes in a variety of flavors, and its rich flavors are captivating. However, the original recipe a cheesecake is loaded with unnecessary fats and sugars that can help add the pounds. Rather than avoid cheesecake all together, try this low fat option that skimps on the sugars, but not on the flavors. With this recipe, you can have your cake and eat it too.

In a mixing bowl, add cream cheese, sugar, yogurt, and lemon juicing, beating it with a mixer until it has a smooth consistency and the sugar is dissolved, placing it in the refrigerator once this has been completed. In a separate bowl, combine the strawberries and strawberry preserves. Then, in the food processor, pulse almonds into a crumb consistency. Add the dates, and combine in the processor. Spread the date and almond mixture into two serving dishes, spooning cheesecake yogurt mixture and then the strawberry mixture on top, layering as you please. Allow 2 to 3 hours to refrigerate before enjoying.

Lemon Lime Popsicles

Popsicles are everyone's favorite childhood snack, often invoking memories of blissful and carefree summers. But who said popsicles are only for children? During the hot summer months, and a popsicle can be just the thing you need to cool yourself down, and relax by the pool. Store-bought popsicles can be full of extra sugars and chemicals to make them look and taste perfect. However, you do not need any of that extra in your body. Homemade popsicles are easy, fun, and delicious.

To make lemon lime popsicles, all you need is agave nectar, lemons, limes, and apple or white grape juice. Juice the lemons and limes, and combine with the juice and sweetener. Pour the mixture into popsicle molds of plastic cups, inserting popsicle sticks and sticking them into the freezer. It should take about 4 hours to freeze, and then you have a quick easy snack you can grab on the go.

Homemade Nutella

Unless you have been living under a rock, you have tried or heard about the phenomenon that is Nutella. It is a hazelnut chocolate spread that can be added to any food, and take it to another level of taste. However, it is full of fats and sugars that are unflattering for your waistline. But like most of the snacks in this book, you do not have to miss out on the hype. By using all natural whole food ingredients, you can enjoy Nutella while protecting your diet.

Heat your oven to 275 degrees, and spread the hazelnuts across a cookie sheet, roasting them for 15 minutes. After this time, you can wrap the hazelnuts in a towel to cool for ten minutes. rubbing the skins off of the hazelnuts with the towel. In a pan, add chocolate chips, milk, honey, and salt and heat and stir until melted. Pulse hazelnuts in a food processor until they have a butter like consistency, and then add the chocolate mixture, combining the two together. Put the mixture in a container and refrigerate in order to thicken before eating.

Honey Almond Popcorn

Popcorn is one of the world's favorite movie time snacks, and no movie night can be complete without it. But the low fat popcorn bags you can buy at the store are often bland, and lack the flavor to really capture your taste buds. Instead of suffering through healthy bland popcorn, use this recipe to take your popcorn to the next level without adding calories.

This recipe uses Skinny Girls brand of low fat popcorn, but any brand of low fat popcorn that you have will work fine. Pop the popcorn according to the instructions, and add the popcorn and dry roasted almonds into a large bowl. Sprinkle cinnamon and chili powder over the popcorn, and then pour honey over the top. Gently mix the popcorn together, getting everything combined and coated. Enjoy!

Banana Ice Cream

Ice cream has long been one of the guilty pleasures of many dieters. On cheat days, people flock to their nearest creamery to get their favorite flavors. But why should ice cream be limited to cheat days? With this easy one ingredient banana ice cream, you can get your icy creamy fix without breaking your diet.

Peel your bananas, and slice them into thick slices. Then, you should lay them out on a plate and allow them to freeze for at least two hours. Then place them in the blender, and blend them into a thick consistency. You can then eat it right away, which is recommended, or put it in a lidded container and store it in the freezer until you are ready to eat it.

Pretzel Snack Stack

When you are at work, and looking for a quick snack for after school for both you and your kids, the pretzel snack stack can be a satisfying snack. It combines the salt, sweet, and fruity in one snack, delivering layers of flavor and texture. You won't be disappointed with this updated version of a classic snack.

The only ingredients that you will need are whole wheat pretzel twists, peanut butter, banana slices, and mini dark chocolate chips. The process of making this snack is a serious of layering pretzels, peanut butter, banana slices, and chocolate chips. Continue this layering with four to five layers for a perfect snack.

Chapter 4 – Decadent Food Snacks

Baked Onion Rings

When we go to hamburger restaurants, one of the most prominent sides that can be found are onion rings. They are delicious breaded goodies, but are not good for your diet or your waistline. But the theme of this book has been to bring the unhealthy to the healthy, and these onion rings are no different By changing few details of the recipe, and baking instead of frying these, you can easily keep onion rings in your diet.

In a bowl, you will need to combine whole wheat bread crumbs, flour, salt, pepper, and baking powder. Next, separate onion slices into individual rings and dip into the flour mixture, ensuring an even and full coating. In another bowl, combine milk and egg whites, and combine with the leftover flour mixture. Dip the onions back into this mixture, and place them on a cookie sheet. Drizzle with olive oil, and bake for 10 minutes at 400 degrees, flip, and then cook for an additional 10 to 15 minutes.

Spicy Pumpkin Hummus

Hummus is one of the best foods for you, and can be extremely versatile when it comes to flavors and tastes. In this recipe, just in time for the fall season, a spicy pumpkin hummus will provide a great pick me up for any day. It can be perfect for parties, get togethers or just a snack for one.

It is extremely easy to make this hummus. Combine pumpkin puree, minced garlic, chopped cilantro, Tahini, lime juice, extra virgin olive oil, allspice, cumin, chili powder, red pepper flakes and salt in a food processor, and blend. Pour into a bowl, and refrigerate for 2 to 8 hours before serving.

Black Bean Flautas

Black bean flautas are very much like the taquitos that many people buy in the stores or in frozen food sections. They can be delicious, but because they are often fried, they can be full of unnecessary oils an fats. In order to reduce this unnecessary junk, follow this recipe's and keep your taquitos.

The first step is to combine black beans, cheese, green chilies, cumin, chili powder, black pepper, and salt. Divide the mixture evenly onto the flat tortillas, and then roll tightly. Brush the rolled tortillas with olive oil and place on parchment paper lined baking sheet. Bake in the oven for 25 minutes at 350 degrees until the flautas are crispy, and serve.

Lean Teriyaki Meatballs

One of the most popular trends in food today, is the fusion of different food types. In the case of the lean teriyaki meatballs, you can combine Italian and Asian style foods, for one healthy and delicious snack that can easily be made into a meal for a quick fix.

In a bowl, combine the teriyaki sauce by combining soy sauce, honey, and mirin, mixing until the honey is melted. In another bowl, soak break in milk, and then squeeze out the milk. In yet another bowl, mix beef, egg, salt, pepper, sesame seeds, sesame oil, onions and soaked break until they are fully combined. Take the meat and form small balls, placing them in a skillet with a small layer of olive oil to brown the meatballs. Add the teriyaki sauce into the pan, and cook for another few minutes. Garnish with sesame seeds, and enjoy!

Cinnamon Pita Chips

One of the most common guilty pleasures and bad eating habits of dieters are potato chips. They satisfy the needs for a salty treat, and are addicting once you begin to eat them. But they are one of the worst snacks you can add to your diet. Instead of eating potato chips, you can easily make these cinnamon pita chips. The cinnamon flavor can easily be changed for any other flavor you are craving.

You can buy whole wheat pitas from most grocery stores, and will only need honey and cinnamon to complete the snack. Cut the pitas into eighths, and spread them on a single layer on a cookie sheet, pushing them as close as possible. Drizzle honey of the pita slices, and finish with a sprinkling of cinnamon. Bake for 350 degrees for 15 minutes, and you are finished!

Conclusion

Throughout this book, we hoped to accomplish several things. The first of which, was to provide readers with a list of snack ideas and recipes that will be delicious, as well as nutritious. Snacking is an important part of any healthy diet. Most nutritionists and diet experts agree that the best way to eat everyday is to have three main meals a day, which are breakfast, lunch, and dinner, as well as two to three snacks during the day in between meals. Your major meals should not be made as large as you ate before. Portion control is key, and maximizing the vitamins and minerals in your food versus the sugars and sodium in it are the most important things to consider.

Snacks are an important part of your daily diet. The point of any snack is to give you the energy and fuel that you need in order to get you through until the next major meal. But through this book, we hope that you will have learned that snacks do not need to be boring, or bland. There is a world of snacks that is so much more than just a bag of chips or carrots. Your snacks can be nutritious, yet satisfying. Most of the snacks that we went over in this book have been easy to make, not requiring many ingredients, and being able to be easily adapted to any different flavor profile.

We went over four main groups of snacks – vegetable based, fruit based, desserts, and decadent meals made healthy. Each one of these categories has recipes that are made to suit particular tastes and cravings. Vegetable snacks can be difficult for many people. Many people find vegetables to be too disgusting to eat, but the recipes for yam fries, and spinach artichoke dip, which are both healthy and delicious, can be made in order to get those vegetables back into your diet, while fooling your body into liking the flavors. Fruit snacks are always easier to eat, but must be paired with the right things in order to maximize nutrition. Fruits have a lot of natural sugar which can disrupt the rest of your diet easily. However, recipes like the peanut butter yogurt dip and the baked apple chips will take the goodness of fruits, and accentuate the nutrition, and minimize the risk of eating too much sugar.

The next chapter focused on desserts. Desserts are oftentimes the bane of people's diets. They can be too difficult to give up, and many desserts can end up having as many calories as you are supposed to consume in one day. However, this book has shown you that you do not have to give up cheesecakes, or chocolate popcorn, rather you can adapt them to be healthy and retain their sinfully sweet nature. Finally, we discussed how to take larger meals and decadent foods, and make them into healthy snack sized portions. You never have to give up onion rings, when you learn how to cook them properly.

More than anything, we hope that you found this book to be informative an enlightening on how to best add new and interesting snacks into your diet. Snacks do not have to be boring, but can be exciting and delicious. Thank you for reading!